The Amazing C Italian Cookbook
Authentic Italian Cooking Without the Bad Grains

Copyright

All Information in this book is copyright to C.K. Media Enterprises, L.L.C. and Developed Life Books and may not be copied from, reproduced or sold without prior written permission.

Disclaimer

The information contained in this book is provided for general information and entertainment purposes only and **does not constitute medical, psychiatric, legal or other professional advice on any subject matter**. The author of this book **is not a doctor and make no claims to be one** and does not accept any responsibility for any loss which may arise from reliance on information contained within this book or on any associated websites or blogs. The author of this book is NOT a licensed therapist and makes no claims to be. To read from here onward, it is assumed the reader has taken the diligence to read this message

The "Fire Lotus" Seal of Quality

DevelopedLife.com prides itself on high-quality content. We are against the trend on Amazon / Kindle of cheap, outsourced content written by non-authors.

Free Supplemental Booklet: Right now you can check out www.developedlife.com/subscribe and receive a free copy of the booklet "**10 Success Techniques to Master Your Life**" for those who desire to create optimal life philosophies. This is an important resource to have alongside this book.

You can also visit the exclusive mailing list for natural health and wellness by going to www.developedlife.com/andreasilver, where you can stay in contact with Andrea personally, and get another cool free book: **"The 20 Most Deceptive Health Foods".**

Contents

- Disclaimer 1
- Introduction 6
  - Understanding Your Gluten Free Venture 7
  - Non Sensitivity Related Benefits 9
  - The Case Against Gluten Free 10
- Appetizers 12
  - Scamorza and Spinach Formato 12
  - Farinata di ceci 13
  - Chickpeas Soup With Bacon 14
  - Pumpkin soup with sausage 15
  - Piadina with Prosciutto and Mozzarella 16
  - Polenta with Gorgonzola cheese 17
  - Fried Zucchini Blossoms 18
  - Bagna Cauda 19
  - Beans and Shrimps Soup 20
  - Arancini di Riso 21
  - Baccalà Mantecato (salt cod spread) 22
  - Gluten-free Focaccia Pugliese 23
- Main Courses 25
  - Asparagus and Ricotta Frittata 25
  - Ham and Mozzarella Casserole 27
  - Pear and Gorgonzola risotto 28
  - Canederli 29
  - Mediterranean Rice Salad 30
  - Pumpkin Gnocchi with Taleggio 31
  - Tagliatelle "Primavera" 33

Penne All'arrabbiata 34

Pasta alla Norma 35

Ravioli with Ricotta, Spinach and Basil 36

Pasta Cacio e Pepe (Cheese and Pepper Spaghetti) 38

Spaghetti al Pesto Siciliano 39

Pasta timballo 40

Parmigiana (Eggplant Parmesan) 42

Rice Pizza 43

Mediterranean Cauliflower Pizza 44

Polpette (real Italian meatballs) 45

Cotoletta alla Milanese 46

Potatoes and Artichokes Casserole 47

Mushrooms and Fontina Crespelle 48

Italian Chicken Salad in Lettuce Cups 50

Veal Involtini with Mortadella ham 51

Red Wine and Sausage Risotto 52

Desserts 54

Gluten free "Cornetti" 54

Budino di Riso (Italian Rice Pudding) 56

"Brutti ma Buoni" Cookies 57

"Baci di dama" Cookies 58

Zabaione with strawberries 60

Chocolate Meringa 61

Tiramisù 63

Salame al Cioccolato (Chocolate Salami) 65

Frittelle (Sweet Fritters) 66

Amaretti (Almond Cookies) 67

Castagnaccio (Italian Chestnut Cake) 68

Torrone 69

Ricotta and Coffee Mousse... 71

Caramel Panna Cotta 72

Final Thoughts 73

A Message from Andrea 74

Introduction

The words "gluten free" and "Italian" sound like two things that simply cannot mix together; as the material composition of Italy is about 70% white carbs and pasta. When somebody is about to begin a gluten free diet, often the most regrettable part about it is seemingly bidding farewell to your favourite pasta dishes.

Well, I have some great news: there are a lot of options to make Italian eating your primary strategy for a gluten free lifestyle. There's now a big industry to create gluten free alternatives to regular pasta. And with that, a great deal of awesome recipe options.

Firstly, understand that not every brand of gluten free pasta is necessarily a "winner". I've been through scores of different makes and styles, and found some that are really good and some that are quite bland. A couple of good brands include Rustichella's and Jovial's, which you may be able to find at specialty organic stores.

You will also need to think about the type of pasta. There are many varieties from strange tasting soy noodles to corn pasta. Stick to what works—and usually that's corn pasta. Brown rice and quinoa based pastas can also be tasty. It's easy to mess up a gluten free Italian recipe with the wrong brand of grain substitute. This could spell disaster for your recipe if it comes out very bland.

Finally, I wanted to mention a little about this book: I do a great deal of cooking and worked for several years in a busy kitchen as a professional chef. Although I no longer work in that area for money, you can still find me cooking my own meals for myself or my children on any given day. Now, as for creating this book, I hired an Italian chef friend of mine from Milano to help compile these. My instructions were clear: only the best, most authentic Italian recipes possible—the ones that she'd prepare in her restaurant or for her family near Milano. With Chef Grazia's help, I'm convinced that this will be one of the more authentic recipe collections for your collection / Kindle library.

Understanding Your Gluten Free Venture

Gluten free dieting isn't for everybody. It can be hard. You need to check the labels of everything you buy, and be mindful about gluten when it shows up in unlikely places.

Gluten is found in certain types of grains—namely cereal grains / wheat. Gluten proteins work a bit like binding agents, affecting the elasticity of dough. The most immediate problem that people face with this protein is **celiac disease** which is a very serious condition in which the small intestine is sensitive to the protein, resulting in inflammation, hyper tension, digestive disorders, and eventually serious complications if it's left untreated.

Where things get a bit murkier is the subject of **gluten sensitivity**. It's possible to have problems with gluten without full-fledged celiac diagnosis. It's hard to diagnose, but studies have found links between gluten sensitivity and anti-gliaden antibodies found in the book. Recent studies suggest maybe 6-8% of the population could therefore have gluten sensitivities[1] (NCBI). However, other studies have placed this number higher, with up to 40% of people carrying the HLA-DQ2 gene which predisposes a person to gluten sensitivity[2] (Cleveland Clinic).

Gluten holds more problems, as well. Studies have linked irritable bowel syndrome with undiagnosed gluten intolerances. Gluten is also linked to disrupting the barrier function of the intestine, which could result in further long-term medical complications.

There have been additional studies that have found links between neurological disorders and patients possessing antibodies against gluten[3].

These studies have resulted in a worldwide gluten free dieting trend. This is often performed by people suffering from a multitude of undiagnosed symptoms that seem hard to verify the origins of. Doctors may now suggest eliminating gluten from your diet for 30 days if you are struggling with mysterious, persistent symptoms. As a result of short-term gluten free dieting, patients have reported effects like:

- The elimination of persistent gastrointestinal problems.
- A decrease in bodily inflammation.
- Lowered blood pressure.
- Increased cognitive performance
- Increased energy levels / decreased lethargy
- Weight loss

One of the arguments in favor of gluten free dieting also relates to the famed paleo dieting craze. Our bodies did not evolve to eat

---

[1] http://www.ncbi.nlm.nih.gov/pubmed/23934026

[2] http://www.clevelandclinicmeded.com/medicalpubs/diseasemanagement/gastroenterology/celiac-disease-malabsorptive-disorders/

[3] http://www.ncbi.nlm.nih.gov/pubmed/8598704

gluten and wheat germ. We would obtain or carbs through sources like nuts and fruits, but not roasting bread. Bread is therefore a fairly "unnatural" component to our diets; a chemical that our bodies were never meant to process.

Non Sensitivity Related Benefits

Besides gluten sensitivities, which are somewhat controversial (I will explain in a moment), there are also some practical reasons to give up gluten, anyway. Eliminating gluten also means **eliminating nasty white pasta and carbs from your diet**. I personally have no gluten sensitivities that I am aware of; however, this is the reason why I still prefer to skip the gluten when possible.

White pastas and breads are known as **simple carbohydrates** or **refined grains**. They are linked to conditions like diabetes, weight gain, fatigue, and inflammation. As soon as you take a bite of white bread or pasta, you are eating a mouthful of condensed **glucose sugar**. Because a white bread is refined—the grains have been crushed into that powdery white flour—your body rapidly breaks down the starches, which in turn enter the bloodstream as sugar, causing a sugar spike resulting in short-term lethargy and long-term medical issues, including increased risk of diabetes and obesity.

In addition, when blood sugar spikes, it will also drop shortly thereafter (resulting in the aforementioned lethargic feelings). This drop in blood sugar also increases hunger levels, which will motivate us to go back to the fridge a little while later and get another fix. **This is why carbs, especially refined grains are so dangerous to dieters trying to lose weight!**

While a gluten free diet won't restrict all carbs (that's a *low carb* diet), what you will be getting are non-refined pasta products that won't have quite the same negative effect. Gluten free pastas and breads all typically use healthful ingredients that won't result in immediate blood sugar spikes.

So, based on all of this information, it would seem that adopting a gluten free diet is a no-brainer, right? Well, as with most things in life, there are always two sides to a story.

The Case Against Gluten Free

It's best to look at all sides of an argument before coming to a conclusion, and something we should take away from the skeptics of gluten-free is that not everybody is necessarily gluten sensitive, and sometimes our own minds can trick us into thinking we are sensitive to something when we are not.

Skeptics, in a nut shell, may point to the follow-up studies of Dr. Peter Gibson, professor of gastroenterology at Monash University. Gibson's earlier rigorous scientific work first suggested undiagnosed gluten intolerances among patients reporting frequent gastrointestinal problems.

Gibson, however, was not satisfied with his original experiments and began a new series of tests that were published in 2011. Patients suffering symptoms like bloating, pain and nausea were again provided diets but with stricter controls and randomized variables to blind the patients about what they were eating and how it may affect their symptoms. Long story short, the end result of the testing was that Dr. Gibson believed these conditions were psychological in nature and not gluten related, at all. That is to say, the **nocebo effect** was at work.

The nocebo effect is an interesting phenomenon that hints at the mind's greater physical power over the body. This is when the mind creates its own symptoms and the body reacts accordingly. One of the most famous cases of the nocebo effect occurred in the 1970s when a man died of a terminal cancer **mis**diagnosis simply because he convinced himself he was ill.

What I believe Gibson's work shows is that *not everybody* is necessarily gluten sensitive. Other studies linking gluten antibodies and sensitivities are still quite valid. However, it does not mean that necessarily YOU have these sensitivities or antibodies in question.

However, if you have convinced yourself that you are indeed gluten sensitive, going gluten-free may indeed cure you of those symptoms; as this is the mind continuing to manipulate itself!

The reason I bring up these criticisms is because, now considering myself a veteran in the health field, I worry about "diet craziness" sweeping people off their feet. I remember one time dining with a lady who started freaking out because she found out the tomato soup the waiter brought her had gluten in it; she proceeded to start becoming nauseous and affected by symptoms which I am certain were entirely in her mind.

I don't think it's good to let this happen to you. Before you jump into any diet, consider the ramifications of it, and like a good scientist—evaluate many different variables. In addition to mental trickery, sometimes sensitivities could be the result of dairy (undiagnosed lactose intolerance), or environmental issues (you are allergic to your rosebushes). This is also why doctors suggest to try out gluten free for 30 days and evaluate your symptoms before making any final determinations.

Nonetheless, going gluten free and testing the waters is not a hard thing to do. With this cookbook, you'll have a very solid strategy for trying the diet out; while never running out of a variety of tasty things to eat.

With that being said, let's continue onward to the recipes!

Appetizers

Scamorza and Spinach Formato

The Italian tasty version of the French soufflé.

1 cup ricotta cheese
3 eggs (slightly beaten)
3 tbs extra virgin olive oil
1 tbs rice flour
1 cup scamorza cheese, (shredded)
3 cup spinach (boiled and drained)

Makes 4 serving

Preheat the oven to 450 F (230 C).

In a bowl combine ricotta cheese, eggs, olive oil and rice flour.

Add shredded scamorza and spinach.

Pour into a greased loaf pan and bake for 1 hour, or until the top is golden brown.

Serve hot.

Farinata di ceci

A very traditional ligurian street food made out of chickpea flour.

2 cups chickpea flour
½ cup water
3 tbs extra virgin olive oil
½ tbs salt
½ tbs pepper
½ tbs rosemary

Preheat the oven to 450 F (230 C).

Mix the chickpea flour and the water in a bowl, stir, cover and let it sit for 3 hours.

Coat the pan with 1 tbs of olive oil.

When the batter is ready, stir it, add salt, pepper and rosemary.

Pour the batter into the pan and add the rest of the olive oil and bake for 14 minutes.

Broil the pan on high for an additional 5 minutes, so that a golden crust forms.

Ground pepper, cut into irregularly slices and serve warm.

Chickpeas Soup With Bacon

The best italian comfort food

1/4 cup extra virgin olive oil
1 onion (chopped)
2 cups chickpeas (drained and rinsed)
½ cup pancetta or bacon (diced)
1 tbs fresh rosemary
Salt and freshly ground black pepper to taste
2 ½ cups vegetable broth
1/3 cup Parmigiano Reggiano cheese (grated)

Makes 4 servings

In a saucepan, heat up the extra virgin olive oil.

Add the onions and gently saute until lightly golden, then add bacon, chickpeas, rosemary, salt, and freshly ground black pepper.

Remove from the heat and with a fork mash 1/2 the chickpeas.

Return to the heat and add the broth and cook for approximately 20 minutes.

Add a spoonful of grated cheese on top of each bowl.

Pumpkin soup with sausage

A creamy and velvety recipe for colder weather.

4 cups pumpkin (peeled, seeded and chopped)
½ cup Parmigiano Reggiano cheese (grated)
6 leaves sage
1 onion (finely chopped)
1 clove of garlic
½ cup vegetable broth
1 cup dice Italian sausage
2 tbs butter
salt and pepper to taste

Makes 6 servings

Melt the butter in a small pan over medium heat.

Add chopped onion and garlic; cook for 2 to 3 minutes.

Add the pumpkin and saute until starting to soften; add the broth and a pinch of salt.

Once the pumpkin is tender, puree the soup using an immersion blender.

In a medium saute pan, brown the sausage for 5 minutes; set aside.

Serve hot and top with sausage, sage and shaved Parmigiano Reggiano.

Piadina with Prosciutto and Mozzarella

An Italian flatbread from the regions of Emilia-Romagna and Marche.

2 cup gluten free flour
2 tsp salt
1 tsp baking powder
2 tbs extra virgin olive oil
½ cup ice water
2 cups aragula
2 mozzarella cheese (cut in slices)
8 slices Prosciutto Crudo

Makes 4 servings

Mix together all dry ingredients into a small bowl; add olive oil and water.

Slowly mix the flour and liquid together until it forms a dough easy to handle.

Knead on a flour dusted surface until the dough is smooth, then cut into 4 pieces; roll out to thin circle.

Heat a large skillet on high heat, when hot reduce heat, brush with oil and place flat bread in skillet.

Turn over and brush with more oil and cook other side.

Fold the piadina into a semicircle and stuff with Prosciutto Crudo, aragula and mozzarella; serve warm.

Polenta with Gorgonzola cheese

A golden-yellow Italian cornmeal made from dried, ground maize.

5 cups water
1 cup polenta flour
½ tbs salt
2 tbs butter
¾ cup Gorgonzola cheese (crumbled)

Makes 6 servings

Bring the water and salt to a simmer in a large, heavy-bottomed pan.

Whisk in the polenta slowly and stir until the water returns to a simmer.

Knock the heat down until the polenta bubbles occasionally; cook uncovered, for 45 minutes, stirring every 5 minutes.

Polenta is ready when texture is creamy and thick; turn off heat and stir butter and gorgonzola into polenta.

Serve immediately.

Fried Zucchini Blossoms

Crunchy and utterly addictive, they are a favorite in Italy.

12 zucchini flowers
12 anchovy filets
1 cup Ricotta cheese
2 eggs, (beaten)
½ cup rice flour
1 pinch of salt
3 cups sunflower oil (for frying)

Makes 4 servings

Brush off the dirt on the flower; stuff the zucchini blossoms with an anchovy filet and a teaspoon of ricotta.

Mix the eggs and rice flour together until smooth.

Heat up the oil in a pot.

Gently coat the stuffed zucchini flowers in the batter; fry the zucchini flowers in batches in the oil until golden brown.

Place them on paper towels to absorb the excess oil, and serve immediately with salt.

Bagna Cauda

Literally translated as "hot bath," this specialty of Piedmont often appears in many Italian homes.

2 cups extra virgin olive oil
8 cloves garlic (peeled and crushed)
10 anchovies
Salt and pepper to taste
1 tbs parsley leaves (minced)
2 cups raw vegetables (endive, celery, peppers and courgettes), cut into bite-sized pieces

Makes 6 servings

In a hot pan, pour olive oil in. When the oil starts to warm up, add garlic and turn the flame down.

Add the anchovies; when the garlic gets light brown, about 5 minutes, add salt and pepper and then turn flame off.

Put the sauce in a fondue pot over a flame.

Serve with the vegetable crudités for dipping.

Alkaline Diet Recipes

Beans and Shrimps Soup

Bring a touch of the Italian countryside to your dinner table.

4 cups cannellini beans (rinsed and drained)
½ cup Parmigiano Reggiano cheese (grated)
6 leaves sage
1 onion (finely chopped)
2 cloves garlic (chopped)
½ cup vegetable broth
6 raw shrimps (peeled)
2 tbs butter
salt and pepper to taste

Makes 6 servings

Heat oil in a large pan; add ½ garlic and ½ onion and stir for 5 to 8 minutes.

Stir in beans, broth, a pinch of salt and bring to a boil; reduce heat, and then simmer for 15 minutes.

Puree the soup using an immersion blender.

In a medium saute pan, heat olive oil; saute the remaining onion and garlic until translucent, then add shrimps. Toss lightly until they develop a bright orange/pink color (3 minutes); set aside.

Serve hot and top with shrimps, sage and shaved Parmigiano Reggiano.

Arancini di Riso

A traditional Sicilian rice ball made with leftover risotto.

4 cups leftover risotto (or boiled rice)
1 cup gluten free bread crumbs
1 tbsp parsley (chopped)
2 eggs (beaten)
2 tbs milk
1 cup Pecorino cheese (grated)
1 cup Mozzarella cheese (finely chopped)
1 cup ham (chopped)
1 cup extra virgin olive oil (for frying)

Makes 20-22 arancini

Stir risotto, mozzarella, ham and pecorino in a large bowl to combine.

Using about 2 tbs of the risotto mixture for each, form the balls.

Mix together the gluten free breadcrumbs and parsley.

Add milk to the beaten eggs and mix well.

Dip each riceball into the beaten egg, then roll the balls in the bread crumbs to coat.

In a wide-based pan, heat olive oil; working in batches, add the rice balls to the hot oil.

Cook over medium heat until golden brown on both sides, 3 minutes each side.

Using a slotted spoon, transfer the rice balls to paper towels to drain. Season with salt.

Serve hot.

Baccalà Mantecato (salt cod spread)

A classic and delicate recipe from Venice.

1.5 lb of dried and salted cod (baccalà)
2 cloves garlic
½ cup of extra virgin olive oil
sea salt and black pepper to taste

Place the Baccalà in a large saucepan and cover with cold water; add garlic and bring to the boil , then simmer for 20 minutes or until the fish is tender.

Drain the fish and keep aside a little of the water, remove the garlic and the skin and any bones, then place in a bowl.

While the fish is still hot begin whipping the fish into a cream, using a wooden spoon and adding a thin slow drizzle of olive oil.

Season to taste with fresh ground black pepper and sea salt.

Serve immediately with polenta or gluten free bread.

Gluten-free Focaccia Pugliese

A simple and traditional focaccia recipe from Puglia.

¼ tbs active dry yeast
¾ cup warm water
¼ tbs sugar
½ cup potato flakes
3 tbs extra virgin olive oil
1/2 tbs salt
2 cups gluten free flour
2 medium tomatoes, (thinly sliced)
¼ cup pitted olives (halved)
1 tbs dried oregano
½ garlic

Makes 6 serving

Preheat the oven to 450 F (230 C).

In a large bowl, dissolve yeast in ½ cup warm water, the add sugar and let stand for 5 minutes.

Add the potato flakes, 1 tbs oil, salt, 1 cup flour and remaining water.

Beat until smooth and stir in enough remaining flour to form a dough; knead until smooth and elastic, about 10 minutes.

Place in a greased bowl, cover and let rise in a warm place until doubled, about 2 hours.

Place 1 tbs olive oil in a 10-in. ovenproof pan; shape dough to fit pan, then cover and let rise until doubled, about ½ hour.

Using your fingertips, make little dimples over top of dough.

Brush with 1 tbs of oil, put tomato slices, garlic and olives over dough; sprinkle with oregano and salt.

Bake for 30-35 minutes or until golden brown.

Serve warm.

Main Courses

Asparagus and Ricotta Frittata

An Italian-style omelette enriched with various ingredients.

2 tbs unsalted butter
½ cup shallots (sliced)
¼ tbs salt
18 thin spear asparagus
5 eggs
¾ cup ricotta cheese
1 tbs fresh basil (minced)
1 cup Parmigiano Reggiano or Pecorino (grated)

Preheat the oven to 425 F (220 C).

Heat butter into a large oven-proof frying pan over medium heat.

Add shallots and cook for 3 minutes until they soften.

Add asparagus and cook for an additional 3 minutes.

Beat the eggs and ricotta cheese together, stir in the basil.

Pour the egg mixture into the pan and cook until almost set, about 4 to 5 minutes.

Sprinkle Parmigiano or Pecorino cheese over the eggs and put in oven until cheese is melted and browned, about 10 minutes.

Remove pan from oven and slide frittata onto a serving plate; serve hot.

Ham and Mozzarella Casserole

Layers of ham, eggs, and cheese for a protein-rich breakfast.

2 tbs extra virgin olive oil
2 cups onions (diced)
8 slices ham
6 eggs
pinch of salt
1 cup Mozzarella (shredded)

Makes 6 servings

Preheat the oven to 450 F (230 C).

Add 1 tbs olive oil to a large pan over high heat; when it just starts to smoke, add onions and cook, stirring occasionally, until they are soft.

Beat the eggs with the salt and pepper and add the onions.

Coat a medium baking dish with 1 tbs oil; in the baking dish, layer ham, cheese and the eggs mixture.

Bake for 30 minutes; serve warm.

Pear and Gorgonzola risotto

A sweet interpretation of a classic Italian recipe.

3 cups vegetable broth
1 cup dry white wine
2 tbs extra virgin olive oil
1 onion (finely chopped)
1 cup short-grain white rice
1/3 cup Gorgonzola cheese (crumbled)
1 ripe pear (halved, cored, diced)
½ cup Grana Padano or Parmigiano Reggiano (grated)
1 tbs butter

Makes 4 servings

Bring vegetable broth to simmer in a small saucepan over low heat.

Heat oil in heavy medium saucepan over medium heat; add onion and cook for about 6 minutes, until the onion start to color.

Add rice and stir until translucent, about 2 minutes.

Pour in the wine, stirring continuously, until all of the liquid has been absorbed.

Add 2 ½ cup broth to rice. Simmer uncovered 15 minutes, stirring.

Add remaining broth if risotto is dry; cook until the risotto is creamy but still al dente.

Mix in Gorgonzola and pear; cook until cheese melts and pear is heated through, about 1 minute.

Turn off the heat; add the grated cheese and the butter, cover and allow to rest for a few minutes before serving.

Cover and allow to rest for a few minutes before serving.

Canederli

A rich Italian recipe of Trentino, in the northern part of Italy.

2 cups leftover gluten-free bread (chopped)
3 cups spinach
2 tbs Grana Padano or Parmigiano Reggiano (grated)
3 eggs
1 onion (chopped)
2/3 cup rice flour
2 tbs extra virgin olive oil
pinch of salt
pinch of pepper
6 tbs butter
1 small handful fresh sage

Makes 4 servings

Cut bread rolls into cubes.

Heat oil in a pan over medium heat, add chopped onion and bread cubes and cook until golden.

Wash spinach and boil in salted water for 5 minutes; drain and squeeze out excess water.

Mince spinach with a knife or food processor.

In a bowl, mix spinach with eggs, onion, flour, grated cheese, salt and pepper; stir with a spoon for 5 minutes.

Shape into egg-sized balls and boil in salted water for about 8 minutes.

Melt butter with sage.

Drain and serve with grated Parmigiano or Grana and melted butter.

Mediterranean Rice Salad

The bright flavors of this Mediterranean recipe make it the perfect dish for summer.

1 cup medium-grain white rice
2 tbs extra virgin olive oil
1 onion (finely chopped)
½ cup black olives
½ cup ham (chopped)
1 hard-cooked egg (sliced)
1 cup cooked green beans (roughly chopped)
1 cup cherry tomatoes
1 small handful fresh thyme
1 small handful fresh basil
1 red bell pepper (finely chopped)
1 ½ tbs salt

Makes 4-6 serving

In a medium saucepan, bring 3 cups water to a boil. Add 1/2 tsp. salt and the rice, cover, and simmer 15 minutes.

Remove from heat and let sit 5 minutes; uncover and fluff with a fork.

In a large bowl, whisk olive oil, olives, onion, pepper, basil, thyme and ½ tbs salt.

Add rice to dressing and toss to combine. Add tomatoes, egg, ham and green beans and toss until well combined.

Serve at room temperature or cold.

Pumpkin Gnocchi with Taleggio

A simple and flavorful gnocchi recipe.

2 cups pumpkin (chopped)
3 large potatoes
1 cup rice flour
1 egg
salt and pepper to taste
2 tbs butter
2/3 cup Taleggio cheese (chopped)
8 leaves of sage
¼ cup milk
½ cup Parmigiano Reggiano cheese (grated)

Makes 4 servings

Preheat the oven to 450 F (230 C).

Place pumpkin on a baking tray lined with non-stick baking paper; bake for 40 minutes or until tender, the discard skin.

Place potatoes in a saucepan of cold water; bring to boil over high heat until soft.

Let the potatoes cool for about 30 minutes, then peel with a small knife.

In a large bowl stir pumpkin and potatoes and mash until just smooth; add flour, egg, salt and pepper.

Mix to form a firm dough; if it's too sticky, add a little more flour. To make the gnocchi, spread some flour on a large work surface and cut the dough log into four equal pieces.

Take one piece and cut it in half; roll the piece of dough into a snake about ½ inch thick, then cut it into pieces about the thickness of a fork.

Bring a large pot of water to a boil, then add enough salt to it so that the water tastes salty; before the water is boiling, add the gnocchi in small batches so they don't stick to each other.

When the gnocchi rise to the surface they're ready, about 3 minutes; using a slotted spoon, transfer gnocchi to skillet and toss to combine.

When all the gnocchi are made, heat the butter over medium-high heat and after 5 minutes add taleggio, milk and sages.

Gently toss the gnocchi in the taleggio cream and serve with shaved Parmigiano.

Gluten Free Italian

Tagliatelle "Primavera"

The best colorful pasta dish just right for Spring.

4 tbs extravirgin olive oil
¾ pound rice or corn tagliatelle
2 tbs salt
½ tbs black pepper
1 onion (finely chopped)
1 large leek (chopped)
1 cup fresh peas
2 cups scallion (finely chopped)
15 pencil thin asparagus (chopped)
½ cup fresh basil
½ cup Pecorino cheese (grated)

Makes 4 servings

In a saucepan, heat up olive oil, then add onion and cook for 5 minutes; ad leek, peas, scallion and asparagus and cook for 20 minutes.

Cook the pasta in a pot of boiling salted water; stir to prevent the pasta from sticking together and cook according to the package instructions.

When it's al dente, drain tagliatelle and put back into the saucepan with 2 tbs of water.

Remove pan from heat; add basil, pepper and Pecorino, stirring and tossing until cheese melts.

Cook for 2 minutes, then transfer pasta to a warm serving bowl and serve.

Penne All'arrabbiata

A spicy pasta made from garlic, tomatoes and red chili peppers.

4 tbs extravirgin olive oil
1 cup whole peeled tomatoes (crushed by hand)
½ onion (chopped)
3 cups rice or corn penne pasta
1 tbs salt
3 medium cloves garlic (minced)
1 teaspoon red chili peppers (chopped)
1 handful fresh basil
1 cup Pecorino cheese (grated)

Makes 4 servings

In a saucepan, heat up olive oil; cook garlic and onions until tender, then add tomatoes and pepper and cook for 15 minutes.

Cook the pasta in a pot of boiling salted water; stir to prevent the pasta from sticking together and cook according to the package instructions.

When it's al dente, drain penne and put back into the saucepan.

Cook for 2 minutes, then transfer pasta to a warm serving bowl.

Sprinkle with the fresh basil and Pecorino and serve.

Gluten Free Italian

Pasta alla Norma

One of the most famous Sicilian recipes and tribute to composer Vincenzo Bellini.

3 medium eggplants
8 tbs extravirgin olive oil
1 cup whole peeled tomatoes (crushed by hand)
½ onion (chopped)
3 cups tubular rice pasta (such as rigatoni)
1 tbs salt
3 medium cloves garlic (minced)
1/4 teaspoon red pepper flakes
1 handful fresh basil
1 cup aged ricotta salata (grated)

Makes 4 servings

Cut eggplants into quarters, then sliced into thin rounds.

In a large nonstick pan heat 6 tbs olive oil for 5 minutes; fry the eggplants in two batches, adding a little extra oil if you need to.

Drain the eggplant cubes on a paper towel to remove the excess oil; add a pinch of salt.

In a saucepan, heat up 2 tablespoons of olive oil; cook garlic and onions until tender, then add tomatoes and pepper and cook for 15 minutes.

Cook the pasta in a pot of boiling salted water; stir to prevent the pasta from sticking together and cook according to the package instructions.

When it's al dente, drain it in a colander and put it back into the saucepan.

Cook for 2 minutes, then transfer pasta to a warm serving bowl; add fried eggplants.

Sprinkle with the fresh basil and ricotta and serve.

Ravioli with Ricotta, Spinach and Basil

Fresh, homemade pasta filled with creamy cheese.

2 ½ cups gluten-free flour
2 pinch of salt
1 tbs extra virgin olive oil
5 eggs
1/4 cup butter
2 cups fresh ricotta cheese
4 cups baby spinach (boiled and drained)
1 cup fresh basil
1/2 cup Parmigiano Reggiano (grated)
5 fresh sage leaves
salt and pepper to taste

Place gluten free flour in a food processor with salt, oil and eggs; pulse processor until mixture resembles dough.

Remove from the food processor and place on a gluten free floured surface.

Knead dough by folding over and turning over and kneading for a few minutes, until the right consistency appears.

Wrap the dough in plastic wrap and cover. Allow dough to rest in refrigerator for at least 15 minutes.

In a small bowl, mix together ricotta, spinach, basil, salt and pepper to taste.

Cut the ball of dough in ½ , cover and reserve the piece you are not using to prevent it from drying out.

Flour your workbench and roll out the dough to almost paper-thin.

Using a round cookie cutter cut the dough; brush each round with water and place about ½ a teaspoon of filling into the centre.

Fold the dough to a half circle and firmly press down the edges.

Bring a large pot of salty water to a boil; before the water is boiling, add the ravioli in small batches so they don't stick to each other.

Using a slotted spoon, transfer ravioli to a large bowl and top with melted butter, Parmigiano Reggiano and sage.

Pasta Cacio e Pepe (Cheese and Pepper Spaghetti)

A traditional recipe from Rome.

4 tbs extravirgin olive oil
¾ pound rice or corn spaghetti or bucatini
1 tbs salt
½ tbs black pepper
½ cup Pecorino Romano cheese (grated)

Makes 4 servings

In a saucepan, heat up olive oil, then add pepper and cook for 2 minutes.

Cook the pasta in a pot of boiling salted water. Stir to prevent the pasta from sticking together and cook according to the package instructions.

When it's al dente, drain spaghetti and put back into the saucepan with 2 tbs of water.

Remove pan from heat; add Pecorino, stirring and tossing until cheese melts.

Cook for 2 minutes, then transfer pasta to a warm serving bowl and serve.

Spaghetti al Pesto Siciliano

Almonds and tomatoes give this Sicilian pesto a deep, rich flavor.

½ cup extravirgin olive oil
¾ pound rice or corn spaghetti or bucatini
1 tbs salt + 1 pinch
¼ tbs black pepper
3 garlic cloves (peeled)
¼ cup blanched almonds (sliced)
½ cup sundried tomatoes
2 tbs capers
¼ cup Pecorino Siciliano (grated)

Makes 4 servings

Place garlic, tomatoes, capers and almonds in a food processor and pulse 3 times to start the chopping process; add the ½ cup oil and pulse 4 or 5 times to create a thick paste.

Add cheese and pulse once to mix in, season with 1 pinch of salt and pepper.

Cook the pasta in a pot of boiling salted water. Stir to prevent the pasta from sticking together and cook according to the package instructions.

When it's al dente, drain the pasta in a colander and dump into the bowl with the pesto.

Toss gently like a salad about 30 seconds until nicely coated and serve hot.

Pasta timballo

The traditional simplicity of rustic Italian flavours.

4 tbs extravirgin olive oil
1 cup whole peeled tomatoes (crushed by hand)
½ onion (chopped)
1 cup pork shoulder (diced)
3 cups rice or corn rigatoni pasta
3 medium cloves garlic (minced)
1 teaspoon red chili peppers (chopped)
1 handful fresh basil
1 cup Mozzarella cheese (cut into small cubes)
½ cup Parmigiano Reggiano (grated)
salt and pepper to taste

Makes 4 servings

Preheat the oven to 400 F (200 C).

In a saucepan, heat up olive oil; cook garlic and onion until tender, then add pork, tomatoes and pepper and cook for 20 minutes.

Cook the pasta in a pot of boiling salted water; stir to prevent the pasta from sticking together and cook according to the package instructions.

When it's al dente, drain pasta and put in a large bowl; add sauce, mozzarella, basil and season the mixture with salt and pepper.

Generously butter the sides and bottom of a medium baking dish with 4-inch sides.

Fill the pan with the pasta mixture, pressing down to make sure the pan is filling up evenly.

Bake the timballo about 30 minutes, then let cool for 10 minutes.

Invert the timballo onto a serving plate and sprinkle with Parmigiano.

Parmigiana (Eggplant Parmesan)

One of the great Neapolitan dishes that has spread across the globe.

6 eggplants
1 cup whole peeled tomatoes (crushed by hand)
½ onion (chopped)
2 tbsp extra virgin olive oil
3 cloves of garlic (crushed)
1 tbs salt
5 cups sunflower oil (for frying)
2 Mozzarella (thinly sliced)
1 cup Parmigiano Reggiano (grated)
Handful of basil leaves

Makes 6 servings

Preheat the oven to 400 F (200 C).

In a saucepan, heat up olive oil; cook garlic and onion until tender, then add tomatoes and cook for 20 minutes.

Slice the eggplants and fry them in the hot oil in batches; when they are browned on both sides, remove them from the oil and lay them on a paper-towel-lined baking sheet and let cool.

Spread a few tablespoons of tomato sauce on the bottom of a large baking dish.

Arrange a layer of fried eggplants, sprinkle with some Mozzarella and a generous layer of grated Parmigiano.

Spread the tomato sauce with basil on top and keep making layers (at least 4); top with tomato sauce and a lot of Parmigiano.

Bake in the preheated oven for about 30 minutes, until golden brown on the top.

Serve the parmigiana warm.

Rice Pizza

An alternative to dough style pizza crusts.

2 cups long grain white rice
4 cups water
1 large egg (beaten)
1 cup Mozzarella cheese (grated)
1 cup tomato sauce
Handful of basil leaves

Makes 6 servings

Preheat the oven to 400 F (200 C).

In a medium size saucepan, add rice and water; bring to a boil, cover and simmer for about 20 minutes, until all water is absorbed.

Set aside rice to cool slightly.

In a mixing bowl, combine cooked rice, beaten egg, ½ cup mozzarella; press mixture into a lightly greased pizza pan and cook for 15 minutes, until the top begins to brown.

Remove from oven and let cool before adding topping.

Spread tomato sauce and basil over the bottom of the rice crust.

Sprinkle over with ½ cup grated mozzarella cheese and drizzle with extra virgin olive oil.

Mediterranean Cauliflower Pizza

Bake in preheated oven for 20 minutes; rest a few minutes before slicing.

A healthy and tasty version of pizza.

1 medium head cauliflower (trimmed and broken into small florets)
2 tbs extra virgin olive oil
1 large egg (lightly beaten)
1 pinch of salt
6 sun-dried tomatoes (drained and coarsely chopped)
1/3 cup green olives (pitted and sliced)
½ tbs dried oregano
1 cup Mozzarella cheese (grated)
½ cup olives
¼ cup capers
1 cup tomato sauce
Handful of basil leaves

Makes 6 servings

Preheat the oven to 400 F (200 C).

Place cauliflower in a food processor and pulse until reduced to rice-size crumbles; transfer to a large nonstick skillet and add 1 tbs oil and salt.

Heat over medium-high, stirring frequently, until the cauliflower begins to soften slightly, 8 to 10 minutes; set aside to cool slightly.

In a mixing bowl, combine cauliflower, beaten egg, ½ cup mozzarella; press mixture into a lightly greased pizza pan and cook for 15 minutes, until the top begins to brown.

Remove from oven and let cool before adding topping.

Spread tomato sauce over the bottom of the rice crust.

Sprinkle over with ½ cup grated mozzarella cheese, tomatoes, basil, oregano, olives and caper and drizzle with extra virgin olive oil.

Bake in preheated oven for 20 minutes; rest a few minutes before slicing.

Polpette (real Italian meatballs)

A classic recipe that always brings rave reviews.

1 onion (chopped)
4 cloves garlic (peeled, cut in half)
1 medium carrot (peeled, cut into several pieces)
1 cup ground beef
1 cup ground pork
¼ cup parsley (finely chopped)
½ cup gluten free bread crumbs
½ cup Parmigiano Reggiano (grated)
¼ tsp salt
½ cup extra virgin olive oil

Makes 20-24 meatballs.

Preheat the oven to 400 F (200 C).

Toss the onion, garlic and carrot pieces into a food processor and pulse until the texture is very finely diced. Set aside.

In a large mixing bowl, briefly stir together the ground beef and pork. Add in the processed onion, garlic and carrot mixture, Parmigiano, parsley, bread crumbs and salt.

Mix gently to combine.

Rub a little olive oil on your hands and form the meatball mixture into balls (the size of golf balls).

Fry the polpette in a large skillet; brown each side of the meatball, gently rotating them every 3 minutes.

Lay the meatballs on a paper-towel-lined baking sheet and let cool; serve hot.

Cotoletta alla Milanese

The most classic Milanese dish: the breaded veal cutlet.

4 cutlets of veal rib
1 cup gluten free breadcrumbs
1 tbsp parsley (chopped)
2 eggs (beaten)
2 tbs milk
5 tbs extra olive oil
1 tbsp butter
1 lemon (cut into wedges)

Makes 4 servings

Mix together the gluten free breadcrumbs and parsley.

Add milk to the beaten eggs and mix well.

Dip each cutlet into the beaten egg; press the cutlet into the crumb mix, ensuring an even coating.

In a wide-based pan, heat olive oil and butter; once the butter has stopped foaming, add the cutlets.

Cook over medium heat until golden brown on both sides, 3 minutes each side.

Serve immediately with wedges of lemon.

Potatoes and Artichokes Casserole

A quick and elegant dish.

3 tbs extra virgin olive oil
3 large potatoes (peeled)
4 large artichokes (chopped)
1 cup Parmigiano Reggiano cheese (grated)
1 medium Mozzarella cheese (sliced)
salt and pepper to taste
1 tbs butter
1 tbs fresh thyme

Makes 4 servings

Preheat the oven to 350 F (180 C).

Fill a bowl with water, stir in the lemon juice, add the artichokes and leave to soak for about 15 minutes.

Boil the potatoes until smooth, then let cool for 15 minutes; slice potatoes.

Drain the artichokes and place them on top of the potatoes;

Grease a baking dish with butter; place the potato slices and a few mozzarella slices in the dish. Season with salt and pepper, sprinkle with Parmigiano and a drizzle of olive oil.

Keep making layers until you have ingredients.

Sprinkle with the remaining Parmigiano and thyme, season with salt and pepper and drizzle with the olive oil.

Bake for about an hour; serve warm.

Mushrooms and Fontina Crespelle

Wonderfully thin, savoury pancakes spread with Italian cheese.

4 large eggs
1 cup rice flour
1 cup half fat milk
1 tbs salt
4 tbs extra virgin olive oil
1 onion (chopped)
1 tbs garlic (chopped)
2 cups mushrooms (sliced)
1 cup Fontina Cheese (chopped)
½ cup Grana Padano cheese (grated)
2 tbs butter
salt and black Pepper to taste

Makes 4 servings

Place the eggs, flour, milk and 1 tbs salt in a bowl; whisk until the batter becomes smooth.

Lightly grease a wide-based pan with butter; pour a ladle full of batter into the middle of the pan and swirl it around; use the back of the ladle to spread it thinly over the pan base.

Check with a spatula if the underside is golden brown (2 to 3 minutes); flip the crespella and cook on the other side, then slide the crespella out onto a clean plate.

Keep making crespelle until batter is finished.

Preheat the oven to 350F (180C).

Grease a large baking dish with butter.

Set a large saucepan over medium heat; add oil, garlic and onion and cook until pale gold.

Add the mushrooms and cook for 15 minutes.

Transfer the mushrooms to a bowl and combine Fontina cheese and half the Parmesan.

Stuff and fold crespelle with the mushrooms mixture; place in buttered baking dish.

Sprinkle with remaining Grana Padano cheese; bake on upper level of oven for 20 minute or until top is golden brown.

Remove from oven and rest for 5 minutes; serve warm.

Italian Chicken Salad in Lettuce Cups

A delightful recipe for hot summer days.

3 cups chicken (coarsely shredded roasted)
1 tbs cup fresh parsley (chopped)
2 tbs lemon juice
3 tbs white wine vinegar
½ cup capers
6 tbs mayonnaise
1 cup Fontina cheese (chopped)
2 garlic cloves (minced)
4 tbs extra virgin olive oil
salt and pepper to taste

Makes 4 servings

Combine the mayonnaise, vinegar, lemon juice, salt and pepper in a blender; gradually add the oil and blend until emulsified.

Toss the chicken, Fontina cheese, onion, garlic, parsley and capers in a large bowl with enough vinaigrette and mayonnaise to moisten.

Arrange 1 small lettuce cup on each plate, overlapping slightly; spoon the chicken salad into the lettuce cups.

Drizzle more vinaigrette over the salads and serve.

Veal Involtini with Mortadella ham

A traditional and tasty Sicilian recipe.

4 cutlets of veal scaloppine
2 fresh thyme (chopped)
6 fresh basil leaves
8 very thin slices Mortadella ham
1 cup Pecorino Siciliano cheese (grated)
2 tbs pine nuts
2 tbs extra virgin olive oil
1 cup tomato sauce
½ cup olives
salt and pepper to taste

Makes 8 involtini

Place the pecorino cheese, thyme, pine nuts, garlic, oil and parsley in a medium bowl; toss together and season to taste with salt and freshly ground pepper.

Lay out one slice of veal; pound with a meat mallet until very thin and cut in two.

Trim one slice of mortadella to fit veal; spoon about 2 tbs of the filling on top of the mortadella.

Fold in the sides of the beef slice; tuck in the end nearest you and roll up the slice.

Secure with a toothpick; repeat for remaining slices.

In a wide-based pan, heat olive oil; once hot add the involtini.

Cook over medium heat until golden brown on both sides, 3 minutes each side; cover with homemade tomato sauce, basil and olives; simmer for 5 minutes.

Serve immediately.

Red Wine and Sausage Risotto

This traditional recipe makes great comfort food for those cold, winter days.

3 cups vegetable broth
1 cup red wine
2 tbs extra virgin olive oil
1 onion (finely chopped)
1 cup short-grain white rice
1 cup Italian sweet sausage (chopped)
½ cup Grana Padano or Parmigiano Reggiano (grated)
1 small handful fresh thyme
1 tbs butter

Makes 4 servings

Bring vegetable broth to simmer in a small saucepan over low heat.

Heat oil in heavy medium saucepan over medium heat; add onion and cook for about 6 minutes, until the onion start to color, then add sausage and cook for 3 minutes.

Add rice and stir until translucent, about 2 minutes.

Pour in the wine, stirring continuously, until all of the liquid has been absorbed.

Add 2 ½ cup broth to rice. Simmer uncovered 15 minutes, stirring.

Add remaining broth if risotto is dry; cook until the risotto is creamy but still al dente.

Turn off the heat; add the grated cheese and the butter, fold in the chopped thyme leaves.

Cover and allow to rest for a few minutes before serving.

Desserts

Gluten free "Cornetti"

The sweet Italian version of croissant.

½ cup butter (slightly softened)
1 cup butter (frozen)
2 cup gluten free flour mix (rice-based or sorghum-based)
1 cup milk
¼ tbs yeast
4 tbs sugar
2 eggs (beaten)
3 tbs icing sugar

Makes 16 small servings

Put 1 cup of flour mixture into a medium bowl with yeast and sugar and blend.

Add milk, eggs and melted butter and beat until smooth.

In a separate large bowl, cut cold butter into remaining flour; add the liquid batter and stir until moistened throughout; cover and refrigerate for 5 hours.

Remove dough from refrigerator and press into a compact ball on a surface covered with gluten free flour.

Divide dough into 2 equal parts; roll each part into a circle and cut each circle into 8 wedges shaped like a slice of pie.

Separate wedges and roll out each wedge through the length of the piece.

Roll up each wedge toward the point and shape into a crescent by curving the edges.

Set croissants on a baking sheet, cover and let them rise at room temperature for 2 hours.

Preheat the oven to 400 F (180 C).

Brush each croissant wedge with egg beaten and place in oven.

Bake 15 minutes or until golden.

Let the cornetti cool down a bit and then sprinkle with icing sugar.

Budino di Riso (Italian Rice Pudding)

One of the most classic North Italian family type recipe for breakfast.

1 cup rice
4 cups whole milk
8 tbs sugar
6 tbs butter
1 tbs lemon zest
¼ tbs ground cinnamon

Make 4-6 servings

Preheat the oven to 450 F (230 C).

In a large bowl mix milk, rice, sugar, butter and lemon zest.

Pour the mix into a greased baking dish.

Bake for 2 hours, stirring occasionally.

Remove from oven and sprinkle with cinnamon.

Let cool down for 15 minutes and serve warm.

"Brutti ma Buoni" Cookies

"Brutti ma Buoni" means "ugly but good". They're a type of almond cookies really popular in Italy.

½ cup + 2 tbs almond flour
¼ cup + 2 tbs sugar
1 large egg white
¼ tbs vanilla extract
small pinch of salt

Makes 20 cookies

Preheat the oven to 450 F (230 C) and grease the baking sheet.

Mix together the almond flour and sugar with a rubber spatula.

In a separate bowl, beat quickly the egg white, vanilla, and salt, then add the almond/sugar mixture.

Drop by heaping tablespoonfuls onto the lined or greased baking sheet.

Bake for 30 minutes; remove the cookies from baking sheets to cool.

Serve with a cup of tea or cappuccino.

"Baci di dama" cookies

Baci di Dama (lady's kisses) are traditional cookies from the Piedmont region of Italy.

1 ¼ cups hazelnuts (toasted and skinned)
1 cup rice flour
½ cup unsalted butter (at room temperature)
½ cup sugar

pinch of salt
1 cup bittersweet chocolate (chopped)

Makes 40 cookies

"Baci di dama" Cookies

Baci di Dama (lady's kisses) are traditional cookies from the Piedmont region of Italy.

1 ¼ cups hazelnuts (toasted and skinned)
1 cup rice flour
½ cup unsalted butter (at room temperature)
½ cup sugar
pinch of salt
1 cup bittersweet chocolate (chopped)

Makes 40 cookies

Preheat the oven to 450 F (230 C) and line two baking sheets.

Put the hazelnuts in the bowl of a food processor and pulse them until very fine, then add the rice.

Cut the butter into pieces, then add sugar and salt to the dry ingredients.

Mix all the ingredients together until the butter is incorporated.

Divide the dough into three equal pieces and roll each piece until it's ¾ inch round.

Cut off equal-sized pieces using a knife, then roll the pieces into little balls and place them on the baking sheet.

Bake the cookies for 12 minutes, and then let the cookies cool on a wire rack.

Melt the chocolate in a bowl set over a pan of simmering water.

Put a chocolate chip-sized dollop of chocolate on the bottom of one cookie and take another cookie, and sandwich the two halves together.

Set the cookies on a wire rack to cool down.

Serve with a cup of tea or cappuccino.

Zabaione with strawberries

A simple Italian custard made with egg yolks.

8 large egg yolks (at room temperature)
¾ cup marsala
½ cup sugar
2 cups strawberries (sliced)

Makes 4 servings

Put the egg yolks, marsala and sugar into a large stainless steel bowl.

Set the bowl over a large saucepan filled with barely simmering water.

Using an electric mixer or a whisk, beat the mixture until it is hot, 4 to 7 minutes.

Put the strawberries in bowls and top with the hot zabaione.

Serve the zabaione immediately or refrigerate it for an hour.

Chocolate Meringa

A crisp Italian meringue cookie with a delicious chocolate taste.

1 ½ cup superfine sugar
1 cup dark chocolate (chopped)
1/3 cup water
5 egg whites (at room temperature)
Pinch of salt
¼ tbs cream of tartar

Makes 20 servings

Preheat the oven to 450 F (230 C) and line 2 large cookie sheets with parchment paper.

Place the egg whites in the bowl of a mixer and whip the eggs on medium speed until mixture forms soft peaks, then add salt and cream of tartar.

Slowly add granulated sugar and continue beating until whites are stiff and shiny.

In a small saucepan, combine sugar and water and stir. Continue to heat the sugar and water to 240 F (116 C).

Gradually stream the hot sugar syrup into your egg whites as they continue to whip on low to medium speed.

Transfer to a large ziplock bag; seal bag, then cut a small piece of one bottom corner of bag and gently pipe out 2 tbs of the mixture through hole onto cookie sheets, forming small well-rounded meringhe.

Bake for 1 hour, until meringhe are firm and dry.

Turn oven off and let meringues sit in oven for 15 minutes; let meringhe cool on sheets on wire racks.

Place the chocolate and the butter in a heatproof bowl; sit over a pan of barely simmering water and allow the chocolate to melt.

Drizzle chocolate on top of meringue and let cool for a while.

Tiramisù

The most famous Italian dessert, made with homemade gluten free cookies.

8 tbs butter
1 cup sugar
2 eggs
4 egg yolks
1 cup gluten-free self-raising flour
1/2 cup ground almonds
1 tsp vanilla sugar
1/2 cup espresso
1/4 cup rum (optional)
2 cups Mascarpone cheese

Makes 8 servings

Preheat oven to 350 F (180 F) and line a baking tray with baking paper.

Beat the sugar and butter together; gradually add the eggs and stir.

Mix flour, ground almonds and vanilla sugar together; add 1/3 cup sugar and butter mixture.

Transfer the mixture into a piping bag with a wide nozzle.

Pipe out finger-shaped batter until all the mixture is used up and put in the refrigerator for 15 minutes.

Bake for 10 minutes or until golden.

Transfer to a wire rack and let the savoiardi cookies cool.

Place the egg yolks and 2/3 cup sugar in a large bowl and whisk vigorously for about 3 minutes or until thickened; gradually add mascarpone and marsala, whisking until well-incorporated.

In a small bowl, put the espresso and rum (optional); dip each cookie into the coffee an place on the bottom of a serving dish.

Once the bottom layer is covered, spread half of the mascarpone mixture on top.

Cover and refrigerate for at least 4 hours; to serve, remove the dish from the refrigerator and dust with a layer of cocoa powder.

Salame al Cioccolato (Chocolate Salami)

Looks like a real salami, but it's a sweet treat.

2 cups tea Amaretti or gluten free cookies (broken into pieces)
1 cup 85% dark chocolate (chopped)
8 tbs butter (at room temperature)
½ cup brown sugar
½ cup cocoa powder
2 eggs
2 tbsp Marsala or Amaretto wine (optional)

Makes 6-8 servings

Chop the cookies and add them to brown sugar, hazelnuts and cocoa powder.

Gently beat the eggs with a fork and add to the mixture of cookies.

Place the chocolate and the butter in a heatproof bowl.

Sit over a pan of barely simmering water and allow the chocolate to melt; add Amaretto or Marsala wine.

Pour the chocolate mixture in the eggs and cookies mixture.

Pour the dough onto parchment paper and work it up to create a smooth, rounded cylinder.

Keep dough wrapped in parchment paper and store in the refrigerator for 6 hours.

Remove the salami from the refrigerator 30 minutes before serving.

Frittelle (Sweet Fritters)

A classic Venetian treat, usually made during the Carnival period.

3 potatoes (boiled)
3 cups gluten free flour (mix of tapioca flour, potato starch, rice starch, rice flours)
pinch of salt
2 tbs baking powder
1 cup sugar
½ cup raisins
1 orange juice
1 lemon juice
1 cup water or milk
5 cups sunflower oil (for frying)
2 tbs icing sugar

Makes 6 servings

Put raisins in hot water for 10 minutes.

Press the potatoes; add sugar, lemon, orange juice, baking powder and flour.

Add the water (or milk), raisins and salt.

Heat the oil in a large pan.

Create balls with two teaspoons and fry them in the oil.

Fry until deep golden brown, rotating the frittelle.

Transfer to a paper-lined tray to drain

Sprinkle with icing sugar; serve hot.

Amaretti (Almond Cookies)

Crisp on the outside and soft inside, amaretti are delicate and easy to make

2 ½ cups almond flour
1 ¼ sugar + 2 tbs sugar (for dusting)
3 egg whites
¼ tbs vanilla extract
¼ tbs almond extract

Makes 30 amaretti

Preheat the oven to 425 F (220 C) and line baking sheets with parchment paper.

Mix together the almond flour, sugar, vanilla and almond extract and stir for a few minutes.

Add the eggs and continue to stir until the dough is smooth.

Place teaspoons of the dough on the parchment paper and dust with sugar.

Bake for 20 minutes or until golden brown.

Cool completely before serving.

Castagnaccio (Italian Chestnut Cake)

The perfect comfort food for cold, winter days.

3 ¼ cups chestnut flour
2 ½ cups water
pinch of salt
½ cup pine nuts
½ cup raisins
¼ cup rosemary (roughly chopped) (optional)
6 tbs extra-virgin olive oil
1 tbs butter

Makes 8 servings

Pre-heat the oven to 200 C (400 F).

Grease a baking pan with butter.

Put the chestnut flour in a large bowl with sugar and a pinch of salt, then gradually add the water to the flour until smooth.

Add the pine nuts and raisins, then pour into pan and sprinkle with rosemary and olive oil.

Bake for 30 minutes or until the surface is dry and cracked; remove from oven and let cool completely.

Gluten Free Italian

Torrone

The classic Italian nougat, very easy to do at home.
1 rectangular edible rice paper (cut in two pieces)
3 cups sugar
1 cup honey
3 large egg whites
8 tbs water
2 cups toasted almond
½ cup toasted pistachios
¼ tbs vanilla extract
¼ tbs orange extract

Make 6 serving

Pour the honey into a double boiler and simmer for 30 minutes, stirring with a wooden spoon.

Put the sugar into a small pan with 8 tablespoons of water and cook until it caramelizes.

Beat the egg whites until soft peaks form and then slowly fold them into the honey and mix.

Add the caramelized sugar and mix.

Add almonds, pistachios and vanilla and orange extracts, then mix again.

Pour the mixture into a rectangular baking pan lined with rice paper.

Cover with rice paper, press and level the mixture with a spatula.

Let torrone cool for 1 hour and serve in thick slices.

Almond and pear soft cake

A luscious cake, loaded with beautiful ripe pears.

8 tbs butter
1 ½ cups sugar
1 cup dark chocolate (broken into small pieces)
3 eggs
1 cup hazelnuts (toasted and grounded)
4 very ripe pears

Makes 6 serving

Preheat the oven to 450 F (230 C).

Butter a flan tin and put a disc of baking paper in the base.

Peel and core the pears.

Mix the egg yolks and sugar until the mixture is creamy, then add ground hazelnuts.

In a separate bowl, whisk the egg whites until they're stiff.

Melt the butter and chocolate together, in a bowl over a pan of hot water.

Gently pour the chocolate mixture into the bowl with the egg whites; fold both mixtures together, using a spatula.

Pour the mixture into the tin; arrange the pear halves on top.

Bake cake for about 1 hour; leave the cake to cool for a few minutes before transferring it to a wire rack.

Serve warm or at room temperature.

Ricotta and Coffee Mousse

Elegant, light and easy-to-make dessert.

2 cups ricotta cheese
1 cup cold heavy cream
1/3 cup sugar
¼ cup instant espresso coffee
1 tbs gelatine powder
3 tbs dark chocolate (shaved)
¼ cup water

Makes 6 servings

Put ricotta in a blender until smooth, then transfer to a large bowl.

Mix together heavy cream and sugar in a large bowl until soft peaks form.

Bring 1/4 cup water to a boil in a small saucepan; remove from heat.

Put 2 tbs of the water with espresso in a small bowl, then mix the remaining water with gelatin in another small bowl until dissolved.

Add ricotta to the espresso mixture and stir for 5 minutes, then add gelatin mixture.

Let the mixture cool for at least 1 hour, then transfer to 6 small bowls.

Refrigerate for about 1 hour; serve with shaved chocolate.

Caramel Panna Cotta

An Italian classic dessert, simple to make at home.

1 ½ cups heavy cream
1 ½ cups milk
¼ tbs vanilla extract
1 cup sugar
1 tbs gelatine powder
½ cup water

Makes 6 servings

Pour milk into a small bowl; stir in the gelatin powder and set aside.

Mix the cream, the vanilla extract and ½ cup sugar in a saucepan; slowly bring to the boil over a medium heat.

Pour the gelatin powder and milk into the cream, stirring constantly for 1 minute.

Remove from heat and pour into six individual ramekin dishes.

Cool the ramekins uncovered at room temperature; when cool, cover with plastic wrap, and refrigerate overnight before serving.

To make caramel, combine the remaining sugar and water together in a medium saucepan; bring to the boil and allow it to cook until it reaches a deep amber colour, then set aside.

Break the seal by inserting a small knife between the panna cotta and the mould; turn onto a serving plate and pour some caramel over each panna cotta.

Final Thoughts

One of the biggest problems we're currently facing is "food by convenience". While not everybody suffers from gluten allergies, everybody CAN suffer from the negative effects of constant, sugary white pastas in our diets. This includes diabetes and obesity.

The convenient food culture is not only why a Big Mac costs two dollars but fresh kale costs six, but it's also how a package of white pasta costs almost nothing, while gluten free alternatives are unfortunately always going to be pricier and at times harder to track down (the tasty ones, anyway).

To resist the "food by convenience" culture is a major part of staying healthy in the 21st century. One way to stay motivated is to remind oneself of how food in the olden days was much harder to obtain. We are lucky we do not have to hunt far and wide across the savannah to kill a gazelle to eat. Therefore, the least we could do is hunt across the exotic supermarket aisles until we can cook the healthy meals we need.

At the end of the day, it will pay off with prolonged health, which means the ability to live a longer life among the people we care about. This is why I care about foods that are gluten free, raw foods, and high alkaline foods. These are all excellent dietary methods to ensure long lasting health.

I hope these recipes will stay useful to you as you embark on your own personal health quest.

A Message from Andrea

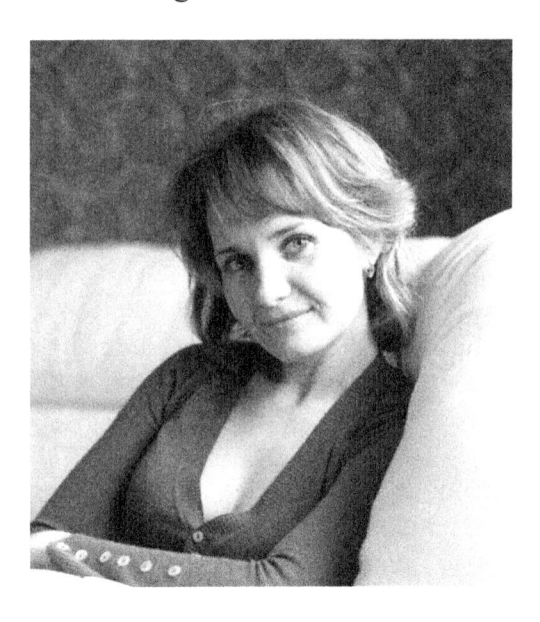

Thank you so much for taking the time to read this book. I hope that this was of some benefit to you.

You can find the rest of the books in this series by checking out www.developedlife.com/andreasilver. You can also reach me personally by e-mailing: AndreaSilverWellness@gmail.com.

A great book to go alongside this one is the first in my *Healthiest Life Possible* series: "*30 Days to Amazing Health*". In this book, I talk about the dangers of downward vortices for our emotions, and practical steps to pull yourself out of a psychological rut--and obtain rock-solid inner-success and health.

Free Gift: At the Andrea Silver page on Developed Life, don't forget to sign-up for my free PDF e-book companion, *The 20 Most Deceptive Health Foods*, which will educate you on the dishonest health food brands and the truly healthy alternatives.

Until next time,
Andrea

Printed in Great Britain
by Amazon